In memo:
Parker Moore,
Lew Cox
11/18/14

Coping with Traumatic Death: Homicide

A book to help you in your time of need

Bob Baugher, Ph.D.

Lew Cox, Victim Advocate

This book is in memory of
Carmon Cox
and is dedicated to those family members
and friends of a homicide victim.

Table of Contents

To the Reader 1

Lew's Story 3

The First Few Days 4
   Shock 4
   The Hospital...5
   Organ Donation..5
   The People around You..5
   The Medical Examiner or Coroner.................................5
   Viewing the Body of Your Loved One 6
   The Funeral or Memorial Service....................................7
   Keeping Organized 8
   The Investigation 9
   Dealing with the Media 10
   Homicide Followed by a Sucicide................................11

The First Few Weeks...13
   Trauma Reactions 13
   Grief Reactions 14
   Medication 16
   Gathering More Information..16
   Charging and Arraignment If an Arrest Is Made 17
   As Life Contines 18

The First Few Months 19
   Preparation for the Trial...19
   Prosecutor's Victim Witness Assistance Program 20
   Pre-Trial Hearings..20
   Plea-bargains..21
   The Trial...22
   The Sentencing 25
   Alternate Charges 26
   A "Not Guilty" Verdict 27

The Grief Process 27
Grieving in a Black Hole 31
Fear 32
If the Murderer is a Family Member or Friend............32
If the Murderer is Still Out There 33
(Re)Visiting the Scene 34
Flashbacks...35
The View of the World Has Changed 35
Reactions of Other People 35
Coping with the Enormous Pain..............................36
Unhealthy Grief Reactions 37
Feeling (or Not Feeling) the Presence of Your Loved One..37
Taking Care of Yourself..38
Re-traumatization and Grief 38

The First Year..40
Unsolved Cases..40
If the Death is a Challenge to Your Faith.................41
Support Groups..41
Deciding to Walk into a Support Group Meeting 42
Bereavement Resources..43
Holidays and Other Important Dates 43

Life after Homicide—The Second Year and Beyond..........45
The Journey 46

Appendix: The Journey Continues...............................48

Acknowledgments 57

About the Authors..58

Discounts for Ordering Multiple Copies.......................60

To the Reader

Someone you know or love has been murdered. The information you are about to read is intended to give you an idea of what to expect after the homicide of a family member or a friend. **It may take all the courage you have to pick up this booklet and read it**. You did not ask for this tragic event to take place in your life. You may be saying to yourself, "I don't want to read anything that will remind me even more of this pain I'm going through."

This booklet was written to help you understand some of what you are going through and to guide you through the homicide investigation. It is not intended to tell you how to feel or to tell you what to do. It is offered as a way to give you some information that may be helpful to your understanding of some of the important issues you will likely be facing. Many people find that they cannot read this booklet all at once. Just read what you can when you can. We have laid out the information in this booklet in an approximate chronological sequence: the first few days followed by the first few weeks, then the first few months, the first year and beyond.

Death by homicide has more elements attached to it than any other type of unnatural death. The subject matter in this booklet comes from direct experience and observation. We are sorry that this tragedy has occurred in your life. We hope that this booklet will be informational and helpful as you travel through the maze of both your bereavement journey and the criminal justice system. To give you a greater understanding of what you may experience, we have included throughout this booklet the personal experiences of co-author Lew Cox following the 1987 murder of his daughter, Carmon. So, at various points throughout the booklet we have placed Lew's story in italics.

1

When someone you love is murdered, your emotions become intensified to a greater extent than you could ever imagine. You may feel as though you have been thrown into a tailspin. Shock, disbelief, anger, denial, and guilt seem to know no bounds. Some people feel a loss of faith in both God and humankind. You may feel stigmatized and suffer a loneliness you have never known, all the while feeling confused and wondering why this horrible tragedy occurred. Overwhelmed and horrified, you may feel that you are losing your sanity. You may feel depressed, impatient with yourself and others, and at times you may feel as though you have lost control of your emotions. The only truth we can tell you at this moment is: **you will not feel this way forever.**

Lew's Story

On August 9, 1987, as I entered my office returning from a six-week missionary trip to the Philippines, the phone was ringing. I picked up the receiver and my son, Darren, was on the other end of the line with words that will echo in my mind forever. With his voice trembling, Darren said, "Dad, Carmon was murdered two days ago." These words, which changed my life forever, are beyond human description. This was the kind of news that happens to other families—not mine. My 22-year-old daughter was shot to death by an acquaintance who then fled the crime scene. She died on an elevator as she crawled to get help. My daughter, whom I rocked to sleep as a little girl when she became sick, whom I taught to ride a bicycle, water ski, drive a car, and gave flying lessons to, was dead. As I stood there, alone in my office, the news put my whole body into shock and disbelief as I cried out, "Carmon! Carmon! Carmon!" My mind screamed, "What am I going to do?" I had to do something, so I picked up a broom from my office and I started to sweep the carpet, saying to myself, "What am I going to do? What am I going to do?" As I dropped the broom and broke down sobbing, the surging emotions gripped me like a vice. Then, suddenly, all my emotions were attacked much like a shark in its feeding frenzy. I had no idea a human being could feel such deep grievous pain.

The First Few Days

During the first few days after Carmon's death my body was in total shock. I was on a collision course with feelings and an experience that was foreign to me. My manner was like a robot as I went through the task of making arrangements for a funeral. The tears and pain and the disbelief that one of our family members was a murder victim was bewildering.

Shock

Right now, you are likely in shock, meaning that much of what has been happening does not seem real. People in shock say things such as:

"I can't believe this is happening."

"It feels like a bad dream—a nightmare."

"I feel like I'm just going through the motions."

"I feel like I'm in a fog."

"It's like I'm on automatic pilot."

"There are times I got lost driving to a familiar place."

"For brief periods of time I catch myself forgetting what has happened—then it hits me all over again."

It's OK to be in shock. It is a normal reaction of your body and mind to the overwhelming events that have taken place in your life. Your job right now--as horrible as it sounds--is to take what comes, one moment at a time and just do what you need to do. As time goes on you will begin to feel less like you are in a fog. This may take days, weeks, or months. When this begins to happen, you may find that the harsh, gut-wrenching reality is beginning to hit you—and it hurts—it hurts more than words can describe.

The Hospital

If your loved one was taken to a hospital, you have probably found out that very little was in your control when you arrived. People made decisions and you had little input. You probably observed that the nurses, doctors, and staff were moving from patient to patient. Activity was going on around you while you sat and waited and waited for information that seemed to take so long to come.

Organ Donation

If your loved one survived briefly, you may have been asked about organ donation. Whatever decision you made was fine. The hospital staff was required to ask you. Your job was to do whatever was most comfortable for you and your family at the time. When an autopsy is to be performed, an organ donation may still be possible.

The People around You

You have a right to have support people around you. Ask yourself the question: "Who do I want to have with me right now?" Then ask someone to find those people. This is a time in your life when you need other people to help with tasks such as, driving you around, taking your calls and messages, assisting with household chores, and so on. Ask people directly, "Will you do this for me?" In addition, find someone who would be willing to keep friends and relatives informed of the latest information. You also have the right to ask someone to help so that certain people will *not* be around you. Do what you feel is right for you at this time.

The Medical Examiner or Coroner

The Office of Medical Examiner or Coroner is responsible for the body and for conducting an autopsy in the case of a homicide, suicide, accident, or unknown cause. An autopsy is a surgical procedure intended to determine the exact cause of death. However, in some cases, the autopsy report may not result in an exact cause of death. You have a right to ask for an autopsy report, but will not be allowed to obtain one until the investigation is complete.

Viewing the Body of Your Loved One

One of the questions for you to consider is: Do I wish to view the body? Research with people who have viewed the body of their loved one indicates that most people later felt that it was the right decision for them. Even though they carried the image of their deceased loved one in their mind, they also felt the experience helped them cope with their denial. Some people choose to view the body in the morgue (although this may not be an option) while other people wait to view in the funeral home. If you choose to view the body, call ahead to the morgue or funeral home to set up an appointment and ask the following questions:

"What is the setting where I will view the body?"

"Will my loved one have any visible wounds?"

"Will I be able to touch my loved one?"

"When will I be able to take possession of the personal effects of my loved one?"

"What else should I know before I come?"

Your goal is to find information to help you cope with the realities you are about to face. It would be a good idea to bring a friend or relative with you so they can view the body or autopsy pictures first to determine if it might be too traumatic for you. When viewing a body, injured parts are typically covered. If there were serious injuries to many parts of the body, you may end up seeing only a small portion of it. The length of time your loved one will remain at the Medical Examiner's office varies from a couple days to several days. Call to find their time estimate, but be aware that other emergency autopsies may alter the timetable. The autopsy must be performed before your loved one can be released to the funeral director.

The Funeral or Memorial Service

Despite being in the depth of despair because this traumatic event has happened, you realize you must collect your thoughts and sort out the many tasks to do. Here is a list to help organize your thoughts about the funeral or memorial service:

1. Have I chosen a funeral home? If not, there are two common ways to do this:
   a. Ask friends and relatives for a referral.
   b. Look up the information under "funeral homes" and choose one near you.
2. Do I want a funeral (body present) or memorial service (body absent)?
3. Who in my life is a trusted, strong support person that can accompany me to set up the funeral?
4. Do I realize that it is OK to compare costs between funeral homes?
5. Does a member of the clergy need to be contacted?
6. Who can take responsibility for notifying family and friends?
7. Who can help me with people from out of town?
8. Because people want to help, what tasks can be delegated?
9. Who can take the task of keeping a record of cards, letters, and contributions?
10. Who can help with writing thank-you notes?
11. Prior to the funeral, do I want a viewing of my loved one?
12. What clothing do I want for my loved one?
13. Will this be a religious or non-religious service?
14. Is the church or funeral home large enough to handle the projected attendance?
15. For the funeral service do I want to order a picture video of my loved one's life? Or can a relative or friend create one to be shown during or after the funeral?
16. Are there pictures or mementos I want to display at the funeral?

17. Who will conduct the service?
18. Are there friends or family members who want to participate in the funeral or memorial service?
19. If there is a funeral, who should be the pallbearers?
20. What type of casket (wooden, metal, cloth-covered) do I want?
21. What songs do I want or would my loved one want?
22. Do I want flowers?
23. If people wish to make donations, which organization should they designate?
24. Should there be a burial, cremation, or above-ground entombment?
25. If there is to be a burial, what type of tombstone do I want? What inscription should go on it?
26. If I want to put an obituary in the newspaper , what should it say? Ask the funeral director for examples.
27. If I want to videotape the service (for people who will not be present), who can do this?
28. Who will take the responsibility to head off the media if they arrive?
29. How will I pay for this?

Keeping Organized

During the first week or so, your home may be in a constant state of activity. People will be stopping by or calling to see if they can help in any way, giving their condolences and concerns. If you find that people are making monetary contributions, consider opening a separate bank account to keep track of the donations and expenses. This can help keep track of the financial records during all the confusion. Also, consider having someone take responsibility for answering your phone and responding to messages.

During the time of the funeral or memorial service and burial or cremation, you may appear to be calm and have everything under control. However, you are in a period of shock. In the midst of all this activity, you may not remember a great deal that takes place. This is another reason to videotape the funeral service. Time will seem to have stopped for you. However, the world will still be spinning around. You want the world to stop so you can let everybody know about your pain--to let them know about the hole in your heart, the pain or emptiness in your stomach, and how this all just doesn't see real—it can't be real. You may want to shake the world and ask; "Don't you care? Someone has murdered my loved one!" You soon will realize that the world is not going to stop for you. No matter how long it has been at this point, here is a suggestion: In the midst of all your confusion it is important for you to sit down and write out *all* the questions you can come up with--even those that have no answers. Then decide the people you might contact for some answers.

The Investigation

The police investigation begins when the first officers arrive on the scene of the crime. The investigation may continue for days; and after the funeral is over (although in some cases prior to the funeral), the police will most likely want to meet with you. They will update you on the investigation and inform you if they are charging someone with the crime. If the police do not have a person of interest or a suspect at that point, they will in all likelihood have questions to ask you. Perhaps you may be able to help them fill in some gaps of the investigation.

You may feel you are being asked to provide a great deal of information, but are being given relatively little in return. This can be a very confusing time for you. The police may be asking you questions about your loved one's friends and associations. They might not be at liberty to answer your questions until after they have completed their investigation. They may withhold answers from you because they might have information that only the killer would know. The police investigation could be at a disadvantage if the murderer was able to obtain knowledge of the case. A murderer running loose could be a family member or a friend of the victim. The murderer could cover up evidence if you unintentionally leak information.

A police investigation is a very complicated and labor-intensive endeavor. It may happen that there is insufficient evidence to arrest anyone and the investigation could be ongoing. The harsh fact is that the longer a police investigation continues, the less likely the murderer will be found. Initially, there may be several detectives working on the investigation. As time goes by, if the leads become exhausted and no one has been charged, there will be fewer detectives working the case. It is very likely that eventually just one detective may be assigned part time to the case. Unfortunately, there may be newer homicide cases the detectives will be required to pursue. This means the investigation of the next homicide case will take priority over your loved one's case. If more time passes and the police do not have a suspect and there are no new leads, then the case may go into the inactive file, however not closed. The police officers you meet may range from seemingly uncaring to warmly compassionate. See if you can find one person in the police department, such as the Case Detective, to help find answers to your questions.

Dealing with the Media

Depending upon the profile of the death, you and your family may have been or are the subject of a great deal of media attention. It is bad enough that your loved one has died--now the TV, radio, newspaper, and the Internet are involved. In addition, many families of violent crime victims report that an added burden to their grief was the way in which the media reported the crime.

One of the ways to protect you and your family from being overwhelmed is to choose one reporter and invite him or her to speak with a family spokesperson. If you feel comfortable with this media person, agree to grant him or her exclusive rights to the story. However, be aware that suspects in a murder case quite often find out some of what the police know from what was released by the press. Unintentional damage to the case could occur if family members speak freely to the media. While choosing one media person and one family spokesperson may not sound like a satisfactory solution, most families who have used this approach have appreciated it. When other media people call or appear on your doorstep (yes, it happens), you can dismiss them with the statement, "Our family spokesperson is speaking to only one reporter and her name and phone number is _____." Or you can state that no one in your family is speaking to the media and refer them to the prosecutor and your lawyer. Victim advocacy organizations have experience in dealing with the media. If you encounter pressure from the media, it can prove helpful to contact this type of organization by going to the Internet and typing "victim advocacy." Your local prosecutor's office can also give you a list of victim advocate agencies.

Homicide Followed by a Suicide

Although murder-suicide is statistically a rare event (approximately five percent of all homicides are followed by a suicide), the effects on surviving family and friends are complex. Here are some possible effects. If this is the case for you, see if any apply:

Anger at the perpetrator for both the homicide and for not willing to take responsibility for his actions

A lost chance at justice for your loved one

No trial

Mixed feelings toward the family of the slayer

The challenge of coping with both the shock of the murder of your loved one and the suicide of someone you knew

Guilt feelings for not having done enough to prevent the tragedy

Because of these complex reactions, we strongly suggest that you consider finding a professional who has a counseling background in grief-related homicide. In addition, as we will suggest later, attending a support group is also an important thing to do. However, be aware that your story will be different from those who are still awaiting an arrest or a trial. Despite this, most family members whose loved one died of homicide-suicide reported that attending a support group was a very valuable experience.

The First Few Weeks

At times during the first few weeks I thought I was going crazy. I desperately needed to talk to a father who also had a daughter or son murdered. I needed to have my crazy feelings validated one way or another. In my vain attempt to find another father to talk to about my loss, I came up empty.

Also, during this period, I was trying to make sense of the confusing maze of the Criminal Justice System. All the while, on top of my grief I was trying to reason with myself how I was going to resume life after Carmon's homicide. All of these things were monumental challenges and demands that in no way were going to go away.

Trauma Reactions

Because of the tragic nature of a homicide it is likely that you are experiencing a combination of trauma and grief reactions. Even though these reactions will be listed separately, you will notice that the lists share some common features. Self-help books on homicide and books on grief can provide you with more detailed descriptions of trauma and grief reactions and suggestions for coping. As you look over the lists of trauma and grief reactions, keep in mind that you may experience all, some, or few of them:

Flashbacks of the imagined murder incident

Intrusive thoughts in which you may feel as if you are re-experiencing the events surrounding the day of the murder

Increased arousal, for example, an exaggerated startle response and difficulty falling asleep or staying asleep

A vivid and persistent image of your loved one

Attempts to avoid anything associated with the murder

Recurring nightmares and dreams, which typically involve themes of rescue, revenge against the murderer, and reunion with your loved one

Fear for the safety of you and your family

As the weeks go by, if you begin to realize that the trauma reactions are controlling your life and making it difficult to accomplish your activities of daily living, you may want to consider counseling to help you sort out these issues.

Grief Reactions

Common reactions following a significant loss include:

Shock

Numbness, feeling dazed, overwhelmed

Shortness of breath

Problems in speaking or talking nonstop

Being unable to cry or crying all the time

Confusion

Feelings of unreality

Hyperactivity--a need to move around or get some fresh air

Dizziness, disorientation

Uncertain who you are anymore

Denial—Things you might say are:

"No, it's not true!"

"This is a nightmare."

"No way."

"I can't believe this!"

Depression

Feeling hopeless

Crying

Sick feelings in your stomach

A feeling of not wishing to go on with life

Anger

> Wanting revenge
> Being frustrated at the investigative process
> Feeling upset that your life has been ripped apart
> Blaming others, yourself, or the person who died
> Experiencing aggravation at not having the support you expected
> Feeling betrayed by someone
> Being irritated by little things, such as idle chatter of people around you

Guilt

> Even though you had nothing to do with the death, you may believe you are guilty in some way.
> Examples of guilt statements are:
> "I did this--I'm to blame--It's my fault."
> "If only I _____."
> "I should've (or shouldn't have)."
> "Why didn't I _____?"

Physical Reactions:

> Feelings of anxiety, heart palpitations
> Loss of appetite or overeating
> Sleep problems
> Fatigue, body aches, feelings of heaviness
> Loss of sexual interest
> Nausea
> Headache
> Chest pains

Concentration and Memory Problems

> Difficulty in following conversations
> Reading problems
> Inattention to detail
> Problems remembering appointments and location of items
> Difficulty at work

Medication

If it hasn't happened already, you likely will be faced with the decision of whether or not to take medication to cope with the recent stressful events in your life. The two most common types of drugs used by bereaved people are those that reduce feelings of anxiety and those that reduce feelings of depression. Either of these might help with sleep problems. It is your decision whether or not to take medications to help you cope. Call your physician and make an appointment to discuss your feelings about taking medication. Here is a brief look at the pro and con of medication use:

For: Because a sudden death is so traumatic, medications help a person cope with the ensuing high levels of anxiety and depression. Medication provides a way to take the edge off the intense emotional responses, thereby permitting the person to work on their tasks of daily living. They may be helpful with sleep problems.

Against: Most medications have side effects. Medications often make a person feel like they are not grounded, but rather floating through the day. Medications mask the true emotional reactions to a trauma. When medications are stopped, the person may still have to deal with bereavement reactions.

Gathering More Information

Some people want to find out as much as they can about the events surrounding the death of their loved one. Other people have no desire to do so. If you are in the first group, you may find that your investigation turned up additional information. This may give you more of a sense of control or even a feeling of hope about the progress of the investigation. For many people, filling in the gaps helps them deal with facts rather than wild speculation. For other people it could produce more frustration as they realize how the crime actually happened. It may happen that you spend time searching for more information and end up reaching a number of dead ends. For people who experience these dead ends, it can be highly frustrating and intensify the pain of their grief. We are not saying, "Don't search for more information." Rather, we are trying to prepare you in case your search does not yield the results you hoped for. In addition, don't forget the earlier warning regarding the potential disruption of the investigation.

Charging and Arraignment If an Arrest Is Made

In most states court rules mandate that, once a suspect is arrested, he or she must be brought before the Court (judge) by the close of the business day following the date of the arrest. At that time this person must be charged or released. In some cases the accused person can be held in jail for up to 72 hours following the arrest. However, if this person is not charged within that period, he or she must be released. Some states have a Grand Jury system[1] in which a six or twelve-member jury reviews evidence before the accused can be brought before court.

The defendant also has the right to a speedy trial within 60 days if in custody (90 days if not in custody) after being charged with a crime. In reality however, rarely does a trial take place within this time period. A defense attorney would have difficulty preparing for a murder case within this time. The defendant, therefore, would likely give up his or her rights to a speedy trial.

When a person is arraigned (brought before the court) on murder charges, you might be surprised to find that the plea they give is "not guilty." Although law does not require a "not guilty" plea at arraignment, a guilty plea on a murder charge at the initial arraignment is seldom entered. This is because, on a charge as

---

1. A jury called to determine whether sufficient evidence exists to warrant a trial of a person or persons accused of a crime.

serious as homicide, the defense attorney is virtually required to review the "discovery" (police/lab technician/forensic expert reports) and discuss it with the accused to determine if there is any plausible defense. Theoretically, only experienced and competent attorneys are permitted to defend murder cases. Those attorneys will invariably find information that they feel will help in the defense of the accused. For example, if the "facts" have any gaps, the defense will maintain that the prosecutor charged an innocent person, and urge the jury to find "reasonable doubt" as to guilt. If there appears to be sufficient evidence of guilt of the murder, the defense will usually try (1) to tell a convincing story that the defendant acted in "self-defense"; or (2) to claim that the defendant had a "diminished capacity" or was "insane" at the time of the murder. After thoroughly reviewing all the evidence with the defense attorney, the defendant could change the "not guilty" plea to a "guilty" plea. If this happens, there will not be a jury trial. The defendant would go before a judge and plead guilty to the charges and then subsequently be sentenced.

As Life Continues

In the context of the arrest of a defendant or an on-going investigation with or without a suspect, your life goes on. Your sleep may be restless and you may wake up dreading to face another day. Financial burdens may increase with the added stressors of missing work, driving to appointments, funeral expenses, and so on. Many of life's activities may seem meaningless. You may feel angry and wish people would leave you alone or you may feel angry because people have gone back to their usual routines. You are expected to go to work or school, pay bills, drive, eat, shower, solve daily problems, and run errands. However, on your mind is the constant, horrible fact: your loved one has been murdered. You wonder how you can go on. But you do.

The First Few Months

During the first few months after Carmon was murdered I found myself investing a great deal of energy in the trial. After eighteen frustrating months of court hearings and continuances, it finally came down to the trial day.

Preparation for the Trial

If someone has been arrested and charged with the crime of murder, then you and your family members will have added challenges. You will undergo an experience that few people ever encounter. You will enter the complicated and confusing world of the criminal justice system. There will be people in this system who have an interest in getting the murderer off or a reduced sentence. The role of the defense attorney is to defend the accused to the best of his or her ability, using every avenue permitted by the federal and state constitutions and case law. The defense attorney is an advocate only for the client and is obligated to have undivided loyalty in protecting the client. On the other hand, the "State" has the responsibility to present all evidence of guilt.

Unless you were a witness to the crime or have information directly pertinent to the crime, you will not play a part in the trial; you will only be a spectator. This needs to be repeated: it is highly likely you will have no part in the trial. The prosecutor's Victim Witness Assistance Program will keep you informed of the trial proceedings so that you may choose whether or not to attend. It could take up to a year or more before the case goes to trial. A capital punishment (death penalty) trial could take as long as two to four years to get started. The first trial date most likely will be changed. Be ready to experience several delays and continuances (continuation of the trial proceedings at a future date). There are many factors that delay the start of a trial. When motion hearings and trial dates change it can be emotionally exhausting for you. Each time there is a court hearing and for each day of the trial, you have to decide whether or not to garner the courage to be in the presence of the defendant. If you are employed, it is important to inform your employer of your intent to attend the court proceedings. Include in your explanation the unpredictability of the court timetable.

The fact that there may be several delays before the case ever goes to trial will put you on a roller-coaster ride with downward spirals, out-of-control dips and curves, and unpredictable stops and starts. The wheels of the criminal justice system move slowly. You may take time off from your job only to come to court to find out the hearing has been delayed. You walk out the door again wondering whether you will ever reach a day when the trial will be over. Even though it may not feel like it at the time, you will reach that day. But not before all of this pushes you to your emotional limits.

Prosecutor's Victim Witness Assistance Program

Most prosecutors' offices or district attorneys' offices in the U.S. have a Victim Witness Assistance Program in effect. This program provides victims and/or their family members with information about the status of the case, answers questions about the criminal justice system, puts you in touch with community resources, and provides emotional support, impact statement information, and court escort.

Pre-Trial Hearings

Before the trial begins you will have gone through several preliminary motion hearings. Pre-trial hearings are held to examine and identify issues and to schedule times to hear motions on those issues. Motions to demand additional "discovery" or to demand interview of witnesses are commonplace. If the defendant made any out-of-court statements to police, the Court must conduct a hearing to determine if the statement was made voluntarily after proper advisement of "Miranda" rights[1]. The defense will often move to suppress physical evidence, claiming improper search and seizure. Both the defense and prosecution usually make motions to exclude witness statements or limit what evidence may be presented to the jury.

Plea-bargains

The defendant may want to plead guilty to a lesser charge before the trial begins. This is called a plea-bargain. The prosecutor's office would then consider the plea offer. They do not have to accept any offer made by the defendant; they can take it right to trial. If the prosecutor's office believes it could be difficult to get a jury to convict the defendant, they may take the plea-bargain offered or offer their own plea-bargain. If the plea offer is accepted, the prosecutor and the defendant's attorney would go before the Court to see if the judge would accept the reduced charge. The defendant would then come before the judge and plead guilty to the reduced charge. In spite of this fact, the judge does not have to accept the plea-bargain or the sentence that the prosecutor and the defense attorney have agreed upon. In some states the courts are bound by a sentencing guideline range as set by the state legislature and cannot go beyond or below that range without finding aggravating or mitigating circumstances. The defendant also can plead guilty to the crime at any time before the trial. If this happens, the trial does not take place and the judge can sentence the defendant at the time of the guilty plea or order a pre-sentence report in order to obtain information that will help determine the sentence. You may find it frustrating that you have no role in any of this process. In spite of this, it is common for someone from the prosecutor's office or district attorney's office to confer with the victim's family about the facts of the plea-bargain offer.

---

1. This refers to the statement required by law that must be recited to a suspect upon arrest: "You have the right to remain silent. Anything you say can or will be held against you in a court of law. You have a right to an attorney...."

The Trial

At this stage you have experienced months of living with the tragic loss of your loved one. By now you have gone through months of motions and pretrial hearings and, as some of the shock of the death has begun to wear off, the pain may have become increasingly difficult to endure. In the midst of all this you receive word that the trial is about to begin.

Jury Selection. The first thing that takes place is jury selection, unless the defendant waives the right to a trial by jury and accepts a trial by a judge only (called a bench trial—which rarely happens). Jury selection normally takes from one to two days. There will be twelve jurors and, on the average, there are two alternates selected. However, a capital punishment case would include four or more alternates. A capital punishment trial could take up to a month or more to select a jury. The average murder trial takes approximately two to three weeks to complete. A capital punishment trial could take several months to complete.

Trial Day. During the days and weeks of the trial, it is likely you will not have an interest in anything except what goes on in the courtroom. The trial will take on a life of its own and will lock you in an emotional roller coaster ride more intense than you may have ever experienced. During the trial the defendant will be present and will most likely be dressed to create a positive impression in front of the jury. Being in the presence of the person who has been accused of the murder of your loved one can be one of the most unnerving events in your life. In some cases defendants in court have gloated, smiled, or laughed at the victim's family members. You may see little or no evidence of remorse from this person. During the trial you will frequently see the defendant lean over, nod, and converse with the defense attorney. As you sit there, you may wonder how this person can sit there and have a conversation while your loved one is silenced forever. Despite your feelings about all this, you will hear the judge's reminder that you must not display your emotions while you are in the courtroom. An outburst by family members or friends could conceivably prejudice the members of the jury and cause a mistrial. It may be beneficial to sit in on pre-trial motions to get used to being in the courtroom with the defendant.

The ride on this roller coaster will feel secure as the prosecution presents the State's case. However, the ride will take some powerful emotional dips when the defense attorney presents the defendant's case. As the trial continues, you may develop a distaste for the defendant's attorney. You may be upset that the rights of the defendant are carefully protected when, in fact, your loved one had no rights. You may wonder how someone could defend the person accused of murdering your loved one. The defense attorney has taken an oath to uphold the State Constitution and United States Constitution. However, if the defense does a good job of representing the client and the proper court proceedings take place during the trial, then it is less likely that the appellate court will overturn the case. In other words, despite your feelings toward the defense, you ultimately want the best trial possible in order to head off any possibility of the case being overturned—resulting in a new trial.

If You Are Called as a Witness. If you are going to be called as a witness you will be restricted from talking about the case. In some states the law requires family members who are witnesses to be scheduled in the first part of the trial to enable the family to be present for the rest of the trial. The purpose of witness exclusion from court is to prevent witnesses, prior to testifying, from being influenced by another's testimony.

The Case Is Presented. The prosecution (the state or the federal prosecutor) presents its case including pertinent evidence and witnesses. The State has the burden of proof to convince the jury *beyond a reasonable doubt* that the defendant is guilty of the charges. The defense only has to create *a reasonable doubt* that the defendant did not commit the crime. The defendant is not required to take the witness stand. When both the prosecution and the defense have presented their case, the judge will read the jury instructions pertaining to the law and each side will make a final argument before the jury. Next, the jury will move to the jury room to begin its deliberation. Jurors must return with a unanimous vote to find the defendant guilty. Likewise, the vote must be unanimous to find the defendant not guilty.

Hung Jury. If the jury is unable to come to a conclusion, the judge will declare a mistrial. If that happens, the prosecution will have to make a decision about the case. If the prosecution decides to retry the case, the defendant will most likely (though not necessarily) remain in jail. If the accused made bail for the first trial then this person would most likely remain out on bail for the second trial. However, because bail is typically set so high for a person charged with first-degree murder, it is rare for a person to be released. If the person is out on bail, you may be upset that someone you consider to be a murderer is walking the streets. As difficult as this is and, as long as it takes, your job is to let the legal process gradually move forward, despite the slow pace of its timetable.

Death Penalty Cases. In some states, if the accused has been charged with first-degree murder and has committed a felony in the course of that murder or has killed a police officer or public official, or murdered two or more people, then the prosecutor may seek the death penalty. (Not all states have enacted the death penalty. Check with your prosecutor.) In this case, if a defendant is found guilty of murder in the first degree, there will be a penalty phase of the trial. The same jury will also sit through the penalty phase and make the decision. If the jury does not choose to impose the death penalty, then (in many states), the sentence could be life in prison.

It takes a unanimous decision by twelve jurors to sentence a person to death. If the death penalty is imposed, then the offender will be taken directly to death row. From that point, the wheels of the appellate court will go into motion. When a death penalty sentence is handed down, it typically takes ten or more years of appeals before a convicted murderer is, if ever, executed. Three facts to keep in mind: (1) of the thousands of homicides that occur each year, few murderers receive the death penalty; (2) many death penalty sentences are later overturned in the appeals process; (3) More than 150 men who served on death row were later found to be innocent (often through DNA evidence).

The Sentencing

After months of enduring the trial proceeding, finally one day it will be over. If the accused has been convicted, sentencing will usually take place within 30-40 days. You will have struggled through a homicide trial. You may wonder how you were able to keep your emotions in check during such an ordeal. You are relieved—to an extent. Nonetheless, you are now concerned about sentencing and how much prison time the judge is going to order the convicted offender.

In many states, judges are limited to a sentencing guideline grid mandated by the legislators. (You may wish to check with your Victim Advocate or the prosecutor to review the specific sentencing guidelines in your state.) There is a low, mid, and high range for all types of crimes that judges must use as a guideline. In many states, survivors of a homicide victim have a right to present an Impact Statement to the court. The purpose is for you to have the opportunity, if you choose, to convey to the judge the impact this crime has had on you and your family. You are allowed to display pictures; and the judge may allow you to show a video presentation of your loved one. During the penalty phase in a death penalty case a representative of the family may be sworn in as a witness to be questioned regarding the impact of the crime on the family.

For many people, the period immediately following the sentencing is a high point. With the trial over, the prosecutor shakes your hand and sends you on your way. But then you realize that after all the months of court hearings and proceedings, and with the offender going off to prison, your loved one is still dead. You may feel hurt that the jury or judge gave the murderer a sentence that failed to respect the value of your loved one's life. You realize that no amount of prison time the offender receives, even if the death penalty is given, will bring back your loved one. Unfortunately, each person must face these cold, hard facts and somehow come to terms with them after a murder trial. The questions after the trial now become, "What do I do with my life?" "Where do I put my energy?" For all the months leading up to the trial, your life has been the trial. You may find it very difficult to integrate your life beyond the trial. You may also realize that the criminal justice system did not fix your grief or heal your pain.

Although time was one of my best allies, I eventually came to realize that I could neither rush time nor the grief process. In the weeks and months after Carmon's death all I could do to cope was to remember these important words, "One day (and sometimes—one moment) at a time."

Alternate Charges

In some states, in a homicide trial, the prosecutor, under the law, is able to include into the jury instructions a set of "alternative charges," in addition to the original charges. Examples are: felony murder, second-degree murder, first-degree manslaughter, or second-degree manslaughter. Check with the authorities in your state if they have alternative options. The jury would be instructed to consider the alternative options if they cannot reach a unanimous decision on the original charges. In this type of case the jury would have to come to a unanimous decision starting with the original charges. If they fail to agree with the first set of charges then they would have to drop down to the next set of charges. Then they discuss the reasoning behind the next set of charges until they settle on a decision. If they have to discuss each set of lesser-included charges, the jury could be deliberating for some time. If the jurors cannot come to a unanimous decision on any of the charges then a mistrial would be declared and the State would decide whether or not to retry the case. Ordinarily, the intention of a murder trial is for a jury to find the accused guilty or not guilty.

A "Not Guilty" Verdict

If the jury unanimously decides that there was insufficient evidence presented in the trial to find the defendant guilty *beyond a reasonable doubt*, the result will be a "not guilty" verdict and the defendant will immediately be set free. You and your family will be left with your own feelings about the true guilt or innocence of the defendant. The harsh reality of this outcome is that the decision of the jury is final. For families who believed a guilty finding was a necessary outcome of the trial, the "not guilty" verdict is often devastating. The are often tears and outrage at the verdict. Some family members who have been through this report that it feels as though they have experienced the death all over again. If this has happened, find a way to cope with the intense resurgence of emotions you are experiencing. Suggestions for coping are offered later in this booklet. In addition, consider contacting a person who has been through a similar experience.

The Grief Process

If you undergo the experience of the criminal justice system, the trial proceedings will test your ability to be emotionally resilient. During the months of trial preparation you may be forced to shelve your grief because you are focusing your energy on the rigors of the murder trial. You will have to endure many motion hearings and perhaps trial delays. You will be preoccupied with what the jury's decision will be at the end of the trial. On the other hand, if there is no arrest, you will be in a constant state of anticipation for some break in the case. You may jump each time the phone rings, and you may be watchful of the media for anything that could relate to the case. As a result, it may be difficult for you to concentrate on your grief. You will be moving from the normal life you once knew before this tragedy, down a difficult path of grief, and then on to a new dimension of "normal."

You may not believe it is possible to live on or experience joy again after this tragic intrusion in your life. Please believe that your life, as painful as it is right now, will not always be this paralyzing. Others, including myself, have regained meaning to life after the traumatic murder of a loved one. We will never forget this tragedy. Our lives have changed and will never be the same. It may be hard—even strange—to hear that some survivors of a homicide victim claim that in many ways they have changed for the better since the tragedy happened to them. You may be thinking, "I don't need this kind of life-altering tragedy to cause changes for the better in my life." Please understand that I would not exchange the death of my daughter for all the so-called lessons I have learned about life. However, the challenges that you face time after time may strengthen you when you think you can possibly go no further. I have pushed the limits of pain and emotional depths that I thought not possible to endure. As time passed, I realized that all the challenges that I had to face because of my daughter's murder were at the same time building up a resilience to the despair that could have kept me in a constant state of gloom.

The Family. Murder pulls apart the core of the victim's family. Earlier we discussed the range of trauma and grief reactions.

Each family member grieves differently. Men grieve differently than women and children's grief is different than other family members. Family members may fear being out of one another's sight. Couples and family members may have a hard time communicating because they each are so immersed in their own pain. Children can only grieve to their level of maturity. Their innocence of the world, as they once knew it, has been ripped away. You may notice a distinct change in your children after a family member has been murdered. Infants and preschoolers may become more whiney and unruly. School age children may act out at school and they may naturally fear that they or other family members will be killed. Teenagers may become more impulsive. Yet, they also may become reserved and bottle up their feelings. At the end of this booklet, suggestions will be given for getting help. As much as you can, be there for the children in your family and keep the lines of communication open.

Differences in Grieving. While no one will be exempt from grieving the murder of a loved one, the actual displays of grief that we see in the people around us will run the entire range of emotions. Some people openly express their grief, whereas others may show little or no grief. Many who report attempting to avoid talking about and feeling the reality of a traumatic death later said, "It was more difficult to deal with it later." Therefore, some people in your life may seem as though they are not grieving and are unemotional. Remember that you cannot make a person grieve; and you can't make them grieve like you. Never measure a person's grief by their tears or lack of tears or emotions.

Denial. For a time, denial and silence may seem helpful in reducing the pain of the death. Many people do this for a time as they try not to think about the death, the pain, and the dreadful reality that their loved one is never going to return. Eventually you will be faced with numerous reminders that this event really did take place. For some people the reality of the tragedy may sink in within a few weeks following the death. For others, it takes several months, perhaps a year or more. If you find you are having problems at work because of your grief, it may be helpful to give your employer a copy of this booklet and ask a Victim Advocate to come in to speak with your employer on your behalf. Giving other people in your life a copy of this booklet may also help them understand some of what you are going through.

*I realized one day that my daughter was not going to return and I had to resume life without her. To go on with life without Carmon was something that I couldn't even imagine. I also wanted answers about why this person murdered her. I eventually came to the conclusion that I was never going to know why she was murdered. The question before me then became: "What am I going to do with my life now that Carmon is gone?" I had two choices before me: one negative, one positive. I didn't think Carmon would want me to destroy my life by becoming bitter. I decided that I would eventually turn this tragedy into an undertaking to reach out to others with a similar loss. For a time I was paralyzed in my grief, but I was determined to educate myself in the knowledge of grief and bereavement. I read books. I talked with people. I allowed myself to feel the full range of emotions. With a few steps forward and a few steps backward, my life started to change in ways I never thought imaginable when I began to reach out to others who had experienced a similar tragedy. It was then I could sense healing starting to take place in my broken heart. Right now it may be difficult to believe the words I am going to say to you next: **You will experience many levels of healing.**

Most people report that they never arrive at a point in their loss where they say, "Now I'm healed." You are suffering from a broken heart and your soul has been wounded. You will never forget your loved one. The pain of loss will diminish, but their love will always be with you.

Grieving in a Black Hole

After the trial, you might fall into a "black hole." You feel yourself slipping into a state of confusion and dejection. Your disposition will become confusing to you and others at times and you may think you are going crazy—and, in a way you are—grief is a kaleidoscope of crazy feelings coming and going. You may be entertaining thoughts of retaliation or suicide—or both. This type of thinking most likely is foreign and disturbing to you and those around you. You probably never thought you were capable of thinking thoughts of murder towards someone else. It's hard to say how long you will be in this "black hole." However, in time, you will have the laborious job of climbing out of this "black hole" and you *will* come out of it.

My experience in the "black hole" came after Carmon's slayer's plea bargain was completed I didn't know what a black hole was until that time. In the days following the trial I began to spiral into a place of emotional isolation, yet I was surrounded by people. I started running my life as if it was on a treadmill turning at full speed. I knew people were trying to connect with me but I had too many confusing emotions cascading around me to try to explain to anyone the condition of my life. I thought I should have the capability of controlling my thoughts, actions, and emotions. Instead, I was just surviving from day to day—and, at times, from moment to moment. I realized there was no relief from the emotional grief that continued to torpedo my life. I had to fight an exhausting battle to pick myself up out of this pit of despair. Somehow, in this abnormal world of mine, I had to get my life normalized. Then one day several months after the sentencing, when I noticed I was having a good day, I realized there was a little bit of light at the end of this black hole. As more days and weeks slowly dragged on, I started to climb out of this hole. This black hole would try to drag me back when I would have some bad days. Before long, however, I was having more good days than bad days; and I realized I was winning my battle over this black hole. I also came to realize that my experience in the black hole was my way of acting normal in a highly abnormal situation.

Fear

Fear is a common reaction to sudden death. Examples are fear of:

> Going crazy
>
> Losing control
>
> The same tragedy could happen to other family members or to you
>
> Venturing out into a world that now looks more frightening
>
> Loving someone that much again—avoiding intimate relationships
>
> The future
>
> What people will say about your loved one, your family, or about you
>
> Family members suffering painful grief from this death
>
> People forgetting your loved one

If the Murderer is a Family Member or Friend

Many of the homicides that take place each year in the U.S. involve someone the victim knew. If your loved one was murdered by a family member or friend, you have a number of additional issues that complicate your trauma and grief reactions, the trial and sentencing, and your ability to make sense of a senseless act. Ask yourself, "Who is the best person I can speak with to help me sort out these confusing issues?" If you find that family and friends are not able to help, consider going to counseling to get guidance from an objective source. Or you might find a person in a support group who has had an experience similar to yours.

If the Murderer is Still Out There

   If your situation is one where no one has been charged for the crime, then the bereavement process takes on a different kind of grief management. Families who know that someone has been charged for the murder of their loved one have a place to direct their anguish. If no one has been charged in the case, then the question becomes, "Where do I direct my distress and anger?" You are not able to attach a person with the crime. Perhaps, as noted earlier, you and the police have a suspicion of the slayer's identity; but there is insufficient evidence to charge anyone with the crime. If this happens to be your situation, then you are going to experience a somewhat different set of emotions than those who know someone has been charged with killing their loved one:

   Generalized anger—at the world, at the police or prosecutor who failed to bring anyone to justice

   Hypervigilance—a feeling of always being on edge, in this case being on constant watch for who might be the murderer—the man on the street, the woman in the car next to you, a family acquaintance

   No sense of "closure"—in terms of having the answer to the enduring question, "Who did it?"

   Paranoia and fear—feelings of dread that perhaps the murderer may come after you or a family member

   Failure—feeling as if you had let the person who died down because the murderer has not come to justice.

   Whatever your situation, you might find it helpful to listen to the stories of others with a similar experience at a homicide support group. In addition, it may be tempting to conduct your own investigation without involvement of the detectives. Please understand that this not only can be dangerous, but, as noted earlier, also has the potential to disrupt the ongoing investigation and perhaps alter the collection of evidence, which could be used at a future trial.

(Re)Visiting the Scene

Some people have no desire to visit or revisit the place where their loved one died. Other people have some fear about visiting the scene, while others have decided that they are definitely going. If you are considering a visit, answer the following questions for yourself first:

1. "What are my present emotional reactions when I think about going there?"

2. "Who should I take with me for support?"

3. "What do I expect to happen once I get there?"

4. "Who in the police department can I contact to prepare or assist me in some way?"

5. "How can I take care of myself once I visit the scene so that I will be OK?"

Some people who visit the scene consider trying to find a way that the place can be preserved or commemorated in memory of their loved one. Be aware that whatever you do may not be permanent. For example, you may leave something at the scene only to later find it has been removed. Therefore, try to think through any plans you have in this regard.

If the murder scene was your home or work, do whatever you feel is best for you. Some people report that they never can return to the scene. Others do so immediately, while others do so gradually after a period of time. Find someone who can help you make the best decision for your particular situation.

Flashbacks

It was noted earlier that a common reaction following a tragic death is a replaying of the event—or the event as you imagined it—over and over in your head. This may or may not feel under your control. It can interfere with your ability to concentrate and carry out daily activities. Needless to say, it can be very disruptive. One of the most frequent recurring thoughts is, "What was my loved one thinking and feeling during the injury (or injuries) and at the moment of death?" We typically replay what we imagine was the scene in the last few moments of our loved one's life. Our reactions to this scene may include: worry over how much pain our loved one was in, regret that we were not able to save them or to say "Good-bye," and fear that our loved one's final moments were anything but peaceful. If these thoughts continue to be a problem, contact a counselor who can work with you.

The View of the World Has Changed

When a tragedy occurs in our life, our view of the world changes suddenly and permanently. It looks gray and cold. Yet, the world continues to act as if nothing has happened. If you are like many bereaved people, you have lost friends because they could not handle your loss and grief. In addition, you realize how unfair life can be and that your life has been changed forever. Many people report an increase in family problems during this time. Family issues that existed prior to the murder become amplified. Conflicts between siblings, spouses, parents and children are common. If things feel like they have gotten out of hand, consider counseling with a therapist trained in grief and homicide-related issues.

Reactions of Other People

The reality of the death begins to sink in some time after the funeral period. What we're going to say to you next is not pleasant; but we feel it is necessary to give you this information to prepare you for what may lie ahead:

You may find that most of the people who have surrounded you during this period are leaving you and are going back to their families and their respective lives. As time goes by, many of the people who attended the funeral may not be part of your daily life.

We hope in your case that we are wrong; but it is a common occurrence in the lives of people whose loved one has been murdered. Because murder is such a horrific act, most people cannot imagine it happening to their loved ones. When they see it happen to someone they know, they may try to make sense of it by coming to believe that it must have been something the victim did. These people will find it difficult to be around you and your family because you are a reminder of the worst that can happen. Life will never be the same for you because of this traumatic death. Many people in your life will do everything possible to get you back to your old self. When they find out that the old "you" is gone, some will stay with you, but others will slip quietly out of your life. Nonetheless, in time you will meet and make new friends and develop new relationships. You will.

Coping with the Enormous Pain

Listed below are ways that people have coped with the sudden death of a loved one. Certainly some of the behaviors that involve escape from or avoidance of the harsh reality of the death are unhealthy when used in extreme*. (In the next section, we will describe unhealthy behaviors.)

Coping Behaviors:

Talking with someone who is a good listener

Talking with your loved one

Crying

Sleeping with the clothing of your loved one

Wearing the clothing of your loved one

Reading books related to your loss

Joining a support group and sharing your story with people who have been through similar experiences

Finding a good grief counselor

*Using work as an escape

*Taking time off from work

*Using sleep as an escape

*Imagining that your loved one is away

*Reading books or watching television as a distraction

Unhealthy Grief Reactions

Because the range of normal grief is so broad, only three of the most noticeable unhealthy grief reactions will be addressed:

Anger reactions—that hurt another person or yourself, such as yelling, screaming, and becoming physical. It's OK to be angry, but do not let it get to a point where it becomes hurtful or displaced.

Extreme denial reactions—constantly believing that your loved one is still alive or not mentioning your loved one's name again.

Escape through addictions—alcohol, drugs, eating disorders, gambling, overspending, engaging in risk-taking behaviors

Feeling (or Not Feeling) the Presence of Your Loved One

If you find that you have a difficult time bringing to mind the face of your loved one, it might be helpful to look at pictures or videos and tell stories about the person's life. If you presently find this too painful, give yourself time to ease into the pictures and stories. Some people report that they feel the presence of their loved one. Some feel it constantly while others feel it only once in awhile. Other people report experiences such as a visual, sound, or touch sensation that convince them it is their loved one. It is not clear why some people have these experiences and others don't. The important thing to remember is that these reports are not unusual.

Taking Care of Yourself

Even though you may not feel like it, we urge you to do the things that will help keep you healthy. You know what they are. Please do them.

Re-traumatization and Grief

On the Internet, the nightly news, a television drama, a movie, on the radio, or in the newspaper you may see a similar death, trial, or family reaction. It can be highly disruptive when you suddenly find yourself re-experiencing the events surrounding the death. You may find yourself suddenly crying, feeling angry, empathizing with the family members depicted in the story, or experiencing all of those at the same time. There is a term for these unexpected, sudden grief reactions: *grief attacks*. Be patient with yourself. The fact is, years later grief reactions can still emerge. The difference from the initial grief responses is that people tend to get through these emotional episodes more quickly than they did years before.

When Dr. Baugher asked me to co-author this booklet with him, it took me several weeks before I started writing. At that time it was more than ten years after Carmon's death. Every time I set up time to start writing, I found an excuse to delay it for some reason or another. Once I started writing about the story of my daughter's murder I had to take breaks because I found myself reliving the pain of when I first received the news of her violent death. Putting this life experience down on paper was having an impact on me to a degree that I had not expected. It surfaced pain that I didn't know was still buried in me. It showed me that we never really get over traumatic grief. In spite of the pain that surfaced when I started to write my story, I am pleased that this booklet will help others in their grief of a murdered loved one.

The First Year

Many things took place the first year after Carmon's death. Some things I can recall and other things are a blur. I know I was trying hard to act normal under abnormal conditions. As the months went by with Carmon's continued daily absence, I came to realize that I would never know normal as I once knew it.

Unsolved Cases

Not every homicide case is solved. As months turn into years, it may be hard for you and your family to come to terms with the reality that the murder of your loved one may never be solved. In some cases, both you and the police may have a strong suspicion who committed the murder. Perhaps you see this person often, or once in a while. Or this person lives in another city. However, no arrest can be made without probable cause. At this point, the only thing the police can hope for is a break in the case. They hope that someone will come forward with information about the homicide; and the only thing they can do is wait for that break. However, the hard and cold fact is, in some cases, this break never comes. It is not only especially hard on you and your family, but is also hard on the detectives. Police detectives are in the business of arresting criminals and insuring they go to prison. When a murder case goes unsolved, they take it personally.

You may or may not know the person who committed this crime. A family member or friend may be a person of interest to the police. In this case your emotions will run wild. You may even entertain thoughts of retaliation. As we noted earlier, if you believe that a stranger is the perpetrator, you may frequently be looking at people in a suspicious way. As you walk down the street or shop in a mall, you may find yourself asking, "Is he the one?" or "What about her?" You will ask yourself a thousand times over "Why"? "How could someone so violently, of their own free will, take my loved one's life?"

If the Death is a Challenge to Your Faith

Most Americans maintain a religious affiliation. Some people have no belief in God. When we are struck down like a bolt of lightning with the murder of a loved one, those who have a faith in God often wonder where God was when the murder took place. The unfortunate reality is that there are people living in our world who do evil things. Sometimes family members and friends feel guilty because, despite their religious beliefs, they are feeling grief reactions such as anger at God, depression, hopelessness, and confusion about the meaning of life. On the other hand, some people deny the existence of such feelings because they feel it would be a betrayal of their religious beliefs. If you are struggling with your faith, consider talking about it with a caring friend who understands your doubts, with a clergy person, or through prayer.

Support Groups

There are many people out there who have also experienced a traumatic death of a loved one. Some of these people have taken their tragedy and turned it into a cause to help other people touched by a violent crime. They are there to help you navigate the criminal justice system; or in the case of no arrests, they are there to just be there for you as you search for answers that may never come. They are there to listen to you and support you. These support people are the only people whom you do not have to explain things to, because they have walked or are walking in your footsteps. You will receive information about your state's Crime Victim's Compensation benefits. They can give you a list of therapists who are trained in counseling with homicide bereavement. They truly understand!

It is important for you to believe that you are not alone in your hardship and grief. Sadly, each year in the U.S. there are approximately 14-16,000 people murdered. The good news is that there are bereavement support groups and grass root victim advocacy organizations across the United States. People like yourself, whose loved one has been murdered, organize these groups. When you walk into your first meeting, you will see the faces of people who know the pain of traumatic death. They are there to listen to your story, share their story, and offer help where they can. They can support you through all the ups and downs of a trial. They will listen to your frustration if no one has been brought to trial. They are ready to reach out to you and your family for however long you desire. Call your local prosecutor's office or a Victim Witness Assistance Program to find out what resources are available to you.

Deciding to Walk into a Support Group Meeting

Entering a support group may be a hard decision for you to make. You didn't ask for this tragedy in your life. You may ask yourself, "Why do I need to attend a meeting with grieving people I do not know?" You may come up with all the reasons why you should not sit in on a homicide support group. The fact is, if you take the step to try a peer support group, you may find out that this is the only place you will be able to talk about your crisis, the trial (or lack of arrest), your grief, and your loved one. You will likely meet some fine people whose loved one has been murdered. These folks are the ones who know what you are experiencing because they truly have been there. One suggestion: after you attend your first meeting, do not make a decision whether or not to return until you have attended a second or third meeting. Also, be ready to awaken the next day with (as some people describe it) a type of "hangover" because you have done some hard, but necessary work.

Bereavement Resources

There are self-care books written by people who have experienced the trauma of a murdered loved one. In addition, there are books that can help you understand your grief reactions, those of children, and specific issues such as the death of a spouse, sibling, child, parent, or other loved one. You will find many of them at your local bookstore or library or you can go to: www.centering.org, an organization that offers hundreds of books on grief. Advocacy organizations also carry an array of bereavement books. In some cities there are support groups especially designed for children and for adolescents coping with a death. Call your local crisis phone line, hospital, funeral home, or mental health center for referrals and resources.

Holidays and Other Important Dates

Facing the holidays, birthdays, and the yearly dates (the term "anniversary date" never seems to fit) of the death of your loved one can be very challenging. On the yearly dates of the murder many families find some way to acknowledge the memories that often come flooding back. The first few holiday seasons will of course be a heart-wrenching reminder of past holidays when your loved one was still with you. Many people report that the days approaching the holidays are more discouraging than the actual day.

To this day I cannot remember the first Thanksgiving and Christmas after my daughter's death. All I know is that the first holidays came and went. I remember the second holiday season as a somber time for my family. We went through the motions of the season because we had been programmed how to do it from past family holiday rituals. I recall the dinners and the exchange of gifts as an event with no life behind it. I forced myself to go places and put forth effort towards people around me with a total lack of enthusiasm. One evening, during the second year after Carmon's death, I was at a church play with twenty-five hundred people in attendance; yet I felt removed from the audience in some isolated place. A friend sitting next to me asked if I was all right. I assured him that I was fine when I really wasn't. As our family started to heal from this traumatic event, the joy of the holidays eventually returned. We still missed her (as we do today), but the joy, though somehow different, did return. I discovered that the holidays came and went no matter what state of mind I was enduring. Life just kept happening whether I liked it or not.

The holiday seasons and yearly dates will come and go. However, it will be helpful if you and your family seek ways to face these difficult days because there will be other family members (children and grandchildren) who will need you. Here are some suggestions for coping with these difficult days from people whose loved one has died:

Send off balloons.

Set a place at the table for your loved one.

Light a special candle.

Tell stories of the person.

Sing or listen to a special song.

Create an ornament to hang on a tree or a wall.

Visit a special place.

Write a letter to your loved one.

Buy your loved one a present.

Plant a tree, a bush, a flower.

Say a special prayer.

Make a quilt with the clothing of your loved one.

Change old traditions and begin new ones.

Life after Homicide—The Second Year and Beyond

Sometimes the murderer is a stranger; or the murderer is someone the victim knew. Some victims have put themselves at risk because of their lifestyle. Others were in no risk of harm. No matter what the circumstances surrounding the murder, your loved one did not want to die. Nobody has the right to take the life of another person. Nonetheless, you are coming to realize that the horrendous incident took place and there is nothing you can do to change it. Somehow, you know that you have to pick up the broken pieces of your life and carry on—even though you may not feel like it.

We have seen people walk into the support group meeting who have been emotionally crippled because their loved one was murdered. We have known people who could never imagine laughing again. We have held in our arms people who sobbed, feeling they could not picture themselves ever having a future without that person in their life. However, in time, we have seen these very people transform from deep despair to a new life of meaning. Don't get us wrong. They will never forget their loved one. They carry this person in their heart. Their grieving continues to ebb and flow as the years go by. They still experience the "grief attacks" noted earlier, in which something triggers an unexpected grief reaction. It takes a lot of hard work and courage with steps forward and, at times, steps backward. However, with a good network of support, you will progress to depths of character beyond your comprehension. You are a survivor of life's most traumatic event. Even when you find yourself believing that you cannot make it one more moment, you must believe that you can take another step to make it through this day. Challenge yourself to figure out ways of getting you and your family through this maze of grief. You must believe that you also can survive even when you think you are sinking. Do not avoid your grief. Talk about your grief until you are on top of it. Others have survived this type of tragedy and you can too.

Be patient with and kind to yourself. Recognize progress in your grief when it occurs. When it is not the first thing you think about when you wake up, that is progress. Don't be frightened by this. This progress does not mean that you are forgetting your loved one. As we said before, you will never forget the life your loved one lived. When the death, the murder, and your grief are not the last things you think about before falling asleep, that is progress. When you notice that there are times that you are not thinking about the pain you have been through, that is progress. When you look back on your day and realize there has been joy in it, that is progress. As the time intervals increase when you are not thinking about this tragedy, that, too is progress.

Murder is such a frightening word that we avoid saying it. Instead we may use the term "lost" as in the phrase, "We *lost* our loved one." It is important to recognize the death as a murder. To acknowledge that the person was murdered is to reinforce the harsh truth of what took place. It helps others to know that a crime has taken place in the death of that person. It avoids any misunderstanding how your loved one died.

I do not use the term "loss" when referring to my daughter's death. We did not lose her--she was murdered by the evil act of a murderer.

The Journey

I have been through the journey of unspeakable grief. At times, I did not think I could force another step out of my grieving body. There were times the pain was so deep I didn't want to continue to live. Somehow I kept pushing forward and I was determined not to allow my daughter's murderer to control my life. I cannot change what happened to my daughter, but I will not let her death be for nothing. The greatest tribute I can give

Carmon is to reach out to others. That is one of the reasons I consented to co-authoring this booklet. I hope it helps you in your journey.

In 1987, my daughter's slayer was arrested for her murder and ultimately pled guilty and was sentenced to 17 years to life in the state of California.

You can find a wide range of practical information of victim-related issues by going to the following websites:

www.vcvs.org Violent Crime Victim Services

www.ncvc.org The National Center for Victims of Crime

www.vaonline.org Victims' Assistance for homicides that occurred out of the U.S.

Appendix

The Journey Continues:
The Slayer and Parole Hearings

The Missed Opportunity

A year and a half after the crime, Carmon's slayer was sentenced to 17 years to life. This means, after serving 17 years in prison he would become eligible to petition the California Parole Board to submit a detailed parole plan as to why he should be released. I did not attend a hearing at the Soledad State Prison in Central California until 2004.

Why didn't I attend the hearing when he was sentenced at the Los Angeles County Courthouse in 1988? The deputy district attorney talked me out of it as he thought it would be just too hard for me. I was not comfortable with that decision, but I figured they knew what was best for me. At that time, anyone could put a carrot in front of me and I'd follow their advice. Sometimes there are well-meaning people who think they know what is best for you as an individual and as a family. Since I was talked out of going to the sentencing, it was seventeen years before I had my next opportunity to give an impact statement in the presence of my daughter's slayer. That was just too long.

The Importance of Giving an Impact Statement

Let me state here, as the years have passed, I found myself increasingly disappointed that I allowed the system to dictate this decision for me. It has troubled me that I did not represent Carmon in the courtroom when this man was sentenced. I often wonder what the judge must have thought when he saw no one from Carmon's family in the courtroom. This is why it is so important for me to encourage you to represent your loved one on the all-important day of sentencing.

As I entered the victim advocacy field and watched family after family bravely stand and give their impact statement, I have come to realize how important it is for family members of a homicide victim to be given the opportunity to speak to the sentencing judge and have their word be heard by all present, including the murderer. The prosecutor or the district attorney is representing the state where the crime took place. You are the only representative at the sentencing for your loved one. As a community-based advocate I tell close family members of the victim how important it is to convey to the judge the impact that the crime has had on them and their family. Even though it is an intense and emotional time standing in the presence of the defendant and the judge, in all my years working with families, I have never had anyone tell me they regretted giving an impact statement.

Family Impact

*This crime took place on August 7, 1987. At that time Carmon was 22, her brother Darren 23, and her sisters Laura and Casey, 17 and 16 respectively. In this (2015) revised edition of **Coping with Traumatic Death: Homicide** Carmon would be 49, Darren 50, Laura 45, and Casey 44. I have two granddaughters 25 and 17, and one 7-year-old great grandson. Recently, my great grandson played his first football game. There we all were sitting on the bleachers on a sunny afternoon cheering him on. Carmon was missing. Like the thousands of other events that have taken place with our family over the past 28 years, Carmon should have been there. Even though her name may not come up in general conversation we all feel her missing. Murder in a family is the ultimate loss. The most excruciating experience a parent will have in a lifetime is to bury a son or daughter that has been murdered.*

Thief

The man who murdered Carmon is a thief. In a deadly act that took only a matter of seconds he took away an entire branch of the future of the Cox family tree. With the death of Carmon there is no son-in-law, no grandchildren, no great grandchildren, no cousins, no aunts and uncles. Carmon is only known by my grandchildren because they see the pictures of her in our homes. There is nothing we can do about the event of her death or how the system has affected us; but we can choose to integrate this tragedy into our lives. He shot Carmon six times: two times in the chest and four times in the back as she turned to fight for her life. He has been evaluated with a psychopathic personality disorder. In other words, he is a very dangerous person, and we as a family don't ever want another family to experience the pain we have endured from this man. This is why we will attend all of his parole hearings and give our impact statements to relate how, to this day, we are still affected by the loss of Carmon.

*With God's help I have been able to integrate this tragedy and reach out to others by creating **Violent Crime Victim Services**, an organization that offers direct services to co-victims of homicide. By reaching out to the bereaved it has helped me in my lifetime of mending. You will never get over the loss, but it will get better. That's why it's called "grief work." in my life's work, in tribute to Carmon, there isn't anything I'd rather do than be given the honor to sit with a bereaved family who has lost a loved one through a violent crime. My goal is to give them hope that it won't feel this bad forever; my passion is to give them guidance about the grief and court processes, never telling them that it wouldn't be a good idea for them to attend a trial or give an oral impact statement.*

My Family

The mother of my children and I had divorced many years prior to Carmon's death. I had been remarried at the time, and, sadly, my wife subsequently died from a brain tumor two months after Carmon's death. I have been married now to my wife Suzanne for 24 years. She has been a rock and support system for me. She never met Carmon; nonetheless, Carmon has become an important person in her life. Suzanne is a certified victim advocate and an advisor in our monthly support group system.

The California Parole Hearings Experience

In 2004, I had my first appearance in front of the person that violently murdered my daughter Carmon. It is very difficult to describe in words the emotions that I experienced before, during and after that moment. Seventeen years was a long time to anticipate how I would react when I addressed the parole board commissioner in the presence of her slayer. As I turned off the California highway onto the long driveway to the Soledad Prison all kinds of emotions were flooding me: fear, anger, thoughts of what I would say, how I would react, and what it would be like sitting at the same table looking into the slayer's eyes for the first time.

Entering the Room

Because I had done prison ministry in the past, I was familiar with the prison atmosphere, so I was not intimidated by entering the prison facility. Joanne, a victim advocate, met me at the prison check-in area. She said that she would be accompanying me throughout the day. I was grateful for her presence. After I completed the check-in process, she escorted me into the building where the parole hearings were conducted. The stairway leading up to the second floor and hallway was narrow and creepy, with many layers of paint on the walls. I was taken into a briefing room. After a few minutes a Los Angeles deputy district attorney entered the room to brief me on the hearing protocol. From there, I was escorted to the hearing room where I was introduced to the parole commissioner and his assistant. Also in the room were the judicial assistant and the inmate's defense attorney.

Once we were through with the introductions the inmate entered the room with two guards. He was seated and the guards stood directly behind him. The hearing started immediately. The commissioner stated the reason for the hearing and the *inmate was asked if he was going to speak. He said, "No." The commissioner warned that it would not go well for him if he wasn't willing to talk about the crime. I presumed he was not about to tell the commissioner about how he killed Carmon with her father seated right in front of him. During the hearing the commissioner, however, was able to ask the inmate questions that lead him to talk about the crime.*

My Statement

After the inmate spoke the L.A. district attorney read a letter from the Los Angeles Police Department stating why they did not want this inmate to be paroled. The D.A. then spoke, reading from a detailed list why this inmate should not be paroled. The inmate's attorney spoke next, giving his reasons why the inmate should be eligible for parole. This is standard operating procedure. I was the last person to speak before the break. Joanne was seated at a 45-degree angle from me. The inmate was seated to the front of me and to my left. I had a profile view of him; he would have to turn his head to the right if he was to look at me. Immediately my jaw started to tremble when I began speaking. I continued to speak but I could not stop the trembling. What I had to say was in two parts; first, what Carmon was all about growing up, our relationship, and the distinctive laugh that she had. I mentioned a little quirky thing we had when she was eight or nine and I would get up to make a sandwich. She would say, "Hey, Dad, would you make me a sandwich too?" Then, she would ask me to put a lot of mayonnaise on her sandwich. This was just a little reminder of her innocence, to make Carmon real to the parole board.

As I finished the story at that moment, seventeen years of stored-up emotions surfaced. My jaw froze and I could not speak. It was as if an engine in a car ran out of oil and it seized up. Everything in the room came to a standstill. No one in the room said anything. They allowed me the time to grab my composure and I appreciated their professionalism. There was an institutional clock at the end of the room. I stared at the clock and prayed silently, "Oh God, give me the strength to carry on." I was in that state of mind for about a minute or so, but it seemed much longer. Once I resumed, it was as if the afterburners of a jet fighter flipped on. My jaw stopped quivering and the strength in my voice rose up.

I went into the second part of what I had to say. I talked about the viciousness of the crime that this guy enacted on my 22-year-old daughter. I looked at him in his blue eyes and told him he was a coward for shooting to death my daughter. "You shortened her life and your actions ripped out the heart of her family because you were frustrated with your insecure life. And you are a coward for shooting a woman." I told him, "I do not hate you but I do not ever want you out of prison because it is predictable that you will kill again." I then turned to the commissioners, "This is not about my family or me; we cannot change what happened to Carmon. It is about protecting other families from this man's violent nature." I summed up my statement, "Prevention: This is why I'm here."

My Victim Advocate

What became so clearly important to me during the hearing was realizing the significance of the victim advocate in the hearing room. Even through I have been in the victim advocacy field for years I have never experienced the benefits because my case never went to trial. Joanne was an experienced professional. She knew just how to position herself, not next to me, but behind me and off to the side so I could see her from the corner of my right eye. The placement was perfect and I knew she was there for me. That experience punctuated even more the importance of my advocate job as a silent figure in the courtroom when I'm seated with a family encountering the unchartered territory of going through a homicide trial of a loved one. If you've had a loved one murdered, then I cannot stress enough to you the importance of understanding the value of building a relationship with a community-based victim advocacy organization. Many of these agencies are grass roots, born out of the tragedy of a traumatic death. They have walked in your shoes.

The Decision

After I was through speaking we took a break in order for the commissioners to discuss the case and decide if the inmate warranted being paroled. I returned to the waiting room with the advocate and observed the D.A. snacking on maple bars and discussing the dynamics of the hearing. Within twenty minutes we were summoned to convene to the hearing room. We got seated and the inmate was brought in from his holding cell. The commissioner opened the hearing immediately and informed the inmate that he had been denied parole. The major reason was that the crime was particularly egregious. The commissioner said, "You killed a young lady for no reason. You took a six–shot .38 caliber revolver with you and you shot Ms. Cox six times when her back was turned. We find this act of violence very troubling and at this time we think you are a high risk to reoffend." They elected to give him an additional three-year sentence before he can initiate another parole plan and present it at that time.

I was not supportive of the three-year sentence. I didn't understand the logic of all the incriminating evidence that he is a violent predator and they just give him an additional sentence of three years. Their decision was made and I was unable to debate their decision with them. They thanked me for attending the parole hearing, and I was told my input was very valuable to them.

Since 2004

I have been to four parole hearings; my two other daughters have been to three with me. The girls were 16 and 17 when Carmon died. She was very important to them because she was the big sister and was gone from their lives forever. A picture of Carmon was placed on the table in the hearing room. When they spoke they looked right at him with poignant words that obviously made him uncomfortable coming from two women. After the hearing was over they declared it was a huge relief. My son has not attended any hearings and most likely will not go in the future. I say this to show that each family member must make their own choice on how to deal with this aspect of a murder and the importance of accepting their decision.

My wife attended the last hearing December 12, 2013. Her input was powerful. Because she never met Carmon she brought to the table a perspective from a non-victim living with a man who had a daughter murdered. All these years she has been witness to the pain that still surfaces from time to time. She sees the gaping hole that is always there with the Cox family because of Carmon's absence.

This murderer's last parole plan was the weakest of all of them, but he continues to try and try again. I asked him to concede and forgo his parole hearings and not burden us with the emotional and financial expenses of traveling to California. He demonstrates no remorse and he admitted for the first time at this last hearing that he premeditated the crime. This man has been evaluated as a psychopath by the prison psychologist. He manifests amoral and antisocial behavior. He lacks a true conscience and the ability to love or establish meaningful relationships. During this last hearing the commissioner asked him if he thought about killing anyone else during the two-week time period he was at large before he was arrested. He said, "Yes." For someone who is trying to convince the parole board that he is safe to be released into society you would think his answer would have been "No." He is educated with an engineering degree but his antisocial personality disorder causes him to override healthy decisions. This man has a rage inside of him toward women.

The Future

You can see why we will be at his parole hearings as they come up over the coming years. It is emotionally hard to make the California trips; yet we are willing to put forth the effort and emotional energy to make sure society stays safe from this person. As a family, we've worked hard to continue on despite the absence of Carmon in our lives, to be healthy and not let this person control us by becoming embittered. We have been dealt a hand that we did not choose. He has set a plate at our table that we cannot break. Nevertheless, we will not put the food of bitterness on his plate.

We can't change history, but with God's help we set the bar to live a standard that would make Carmon proud.

Acknowledgments

We appreciate the work of many individuals who read and provided feedback on this book. Their valuable input, based on their own personal or professional experiences, helped to make this booklet a reality. Thank you:

Judge Nile Aubrey
Patrice Baugh
Richard & Arlene Bobb
Peggy Cooper Bowen, Ph.D
Cindi Bramhall
Ken & Shari Capron
Suzanne Cox
Terry Dacca
Vicki Dagen-Hanby
Linda Elliott
Mike & Donna Emerson
Marilyn Evans
Patty Gull
Coleman & Jean Harris
James Horn
Gerri Horne
Susan Lee Howland
Maureen Joy

Juan Kenigstein
Rev. Chaplain Tim Klerekoper
Det. Tim Kobel
Sooyeon K. Lee
Joe & Melva Levick
Courtney May
Bettie Mister
Meghan Munford
Chaplain Dan Nolta
Det. Jim O'Hern
Det. Mike Portman
James Powers
Dick Rutledge
Deborah Spungen
Eleni Teshome
Priscilla Warmbo
Det. Bob Yerbury

Thanks go to Kris Baugher, Bob's wife, and to our publisher Ron Engstrom for their production expertise in preparing this booklet for publication.

Thanks, also, to Shawn Baugher, Bob and Kris's son for the cover photo.

About the Authors

Dr. Bob Baugher is a Psychology instructor at Highline College in Des Moines, Washington. For more than 35 years he has taught a class entitled "Death and Life." He has been a bereavement counselor and group facilitator for people who have experienced the death of a child, sibling, spouse, parent, partner, and friend. Since 1987, he has served on the advisory committee of the South King County Chapter of Compassionate Friends (a support group for bereaved parents). Bob has given more than 700 workshops on coping with grief. Other books by Dr. Baugher:

- *A Guide for the Bereaved Survivor*
- *A Guide to Understanding Guilt During Bereavement*
- *Death Turns Allie's Family Upside Down* with Linda Wong-Garl & Kristina J. Baugher
- *Understanding Anger During Bereavement* with Carol Hankins & Dr. Gary Hankins
- *After Suicide Loss: Coping with Your Grief* with Dr. Jack Jordan
- *The Crying Handbook* with Dr. Darcie Sims
- *In the Midst of Caregiving* with Dr. Darcie Sims

Special Note: This book is now available in Spanish: *Enfrentar Una Muerte Traumatica: Homicidio*. See ordering information on Page 60.

Lew Cox is the founder and executive director of Violent Crime Victim Services, a homicide victim advocate organization located in Tacoma, Washington. This organization is actively working on behalf of, and providing direct services to co-victims of homicide. Lew is an ordained minister and has been a missionary, a pastor and has done prison ministry. He is a Certified Trauma Service Specialist, a Certified Victim Advocate, and a chaplain with the Des Moines, Washington Police Department.

Lew was a member of a team of police chaplains that served a tour of duty during Christmas week at the World Trade Center disaster site. Lew was a chaplain on a law enforcement peer support team during the aftermath of the four police officers who were gunned down in a coffee shop in Lakewood, Washington, in 2009. He has worked with more than 900 families as a homicide victim advocate and has been in over 240 murder trials acting as a court companion for co-victims of homicide. Lew is an active speaker and seminar facilitator on the subject of traumatic grief and homicide. Most importantly, Lew has survived the murder of his daughter, Carmon. His life journey continues to help and guide people whose lives have been forever changed by homicide.

Discounts for Ordering Multiple Copies

2-10 copies	5% Discount
11-24 copies	10% Discount
25-49 copies	20% Discount
50-99 copies	30% Discount
100 or more	35% Discount

Price: $10.00 (U.S. funds) per copy
Add $2.50 postage for a single copy
Free postage for U.S. orders of 2 or more copies

Shipping for Canadian or out-of-U.S. orders
will be billed according to postal rates.

Please allow 2-4 weeks for delivery.

Washington State residents add 9.5% sales tax.

Send Check or Money Order to:

Bob Baugher, Ph.D.
7108 127th Place SE
Newcastle, WA 98056-1325

Or e-mail your order and you will be billed

b_kbaugher@yahoo.com

Pricing and taxes subject to change without notice

If you wish to contact Lew, his email is:
Lew@vcvs.org
Website: www.vcvs.org

Books Prices

A Guide for the Bereaved Survivor .... $ 5.00

Understanding Guilt During Bereavement $10.00

Death Turns Allie's Family Upside Down $8.00
with Linda Wong-Garl & Kris Baugher

Understanding Anger During Bereavement $8.00
with Carol Hankins, M.S. and Gary Hankins, Ph.D.

Coping with Traumatic Death: Homicide with Lew Cox . $10.00

Coping with Traumatic Death: Homicide (Spanish) $10.00

After Suicide Loss: Coping with Your Grief
with Jack Jordan, Ph.D $12.00

The Crying Handbook with Darcie Sims, Ph.D $10.00

In the Midst of Caregiving with Darcie Sims, Ph.D. $10.00

Videos Available

Men and Their Grief $25.00

Men and Their Grief: 20 Years Later $25.00

2-DVD set: *Men and Their Grief,*
Men and Their Grief: 20 Years Later $40.00

Discounts offered when multiple copies are ordered.

Dr. Baugher's books and videos can be ordered via
b_kbaugher@yahoo.com

Prices and Taxes Subject to Change

People have asked us about the book cover photo. It is a picture of lights in a tunnel. In turn, we hope this booklet has offered you some light in the darkness of your life.

Sincerely,

Bob Baugher & Lew Cox